RRT® Board Exam Series

Dominate the Physical Exam Portion of the Respiratory Therapy Board Exam

By Damon Wiseley B.H.S.c., RRT

www.respiratorytherapyprograms.com

RRT® Board Exam Series

Dominate the Physical Exam Portion of the Respiratory Therapy Board Exam.

Table of Contents

Biot's
Cheynne-stokes
Apneustic

Work of breathing
Accessory muscle use
Retractions
Tracheal tugging
Nasal flaring

Thoracic Configuration
Atrophy
Hypertrophy
Barrel chest
Pectus carinatum
Pectus excavatum
Scoliosis
Kyphosis
Kyphoscoliosis

Part 4: Palpation of the Chest
Chest Expansion
Chest Percussion
Tactile Fremitus
Crepitus
Tracheal Palpation
Tenderness

Part 5: Auscultation of the Lungs
Breath Sound Characteristics
Normal Breath Sounds
Abnormal Breath Sounds
Adventitious Breath Sounds

Part 6: Auscultation of Voice Sounds
Egophony
Bronchophony
Whispered pectoriloquy

About the Exam

The National Board for Respiratory Care (NBRC) awards the Registered Respiratory Therapist (RRT) credential to graduates of accredited respiratory therapy programs that meet the following criteria:
1. Pass the Therapist Multiple Choice (TMC) exam high cut mark
2. Pass the Clinical Simulation Exams (CSE)
3. Meet other NBRC eligibility requirements.

TMC exam candidates are given 3 hours to complete the 160 questions. Twenty questions are under review for future exams and will not count towards your final score. The cost of the TMC is $190. The TMC exam consists of a low cut score and a high cut score. Candidates who achieve a high cut score on the TMC exam are invited to take the Clinical Simulation Exam (CSE).

The CSE exam includes 22 questions. Two of these questions are under review for future exams and will not count towards your final score.

Unfortunately, the high cut score is known only to the National Board for Respiratory Care (NBRC) and remains unpublished. The cost of the CSE exam is $200.

One thing we know is missing the cut will cost you an additional $150 to retake the TMC-RRT exam. Failing the CSE is also costly, as the price remains $200 no matter how often you attempt it.

Important note: If you don't make the high cut on the TMC, but pass the low cut you will earn your CRT. However, you may not take the CSE exam until you first retake the TMC exam and pass the high cut mark. Then, you must still pass the CSE to be awarded the RRT credential.

About this Book

Congratulations on purchasing this book and committing to making the high cut on the RRT board exams! Taking the RRT board exams can be an intimidating process for those who are not prepared.

This book aims to increase your exam confidence level by preparing you for the physical exam portion of the TMC-RRT and CSE exams. I've tried to add as much value as possible, while also being careful to not overwhelm you with too much information.

The _MOST_ important tools this book will give to you are:

- ➢ **A thorough review of physical exam terminology**
- ➢ **The ability to connect physical exam findings to specific disease processes**
- ➢ **Recommendations based on the physical exam findings**
- ➢ **Practice exam questions with thorough rationales for each correct and incorrect answer**
- ➢ **Practice questions based on the newest and most current NBRC testing matrix**

Exam Tips

The NBRC Hospital

The patients you will be tested on are residents of a very different and unfamiliar place known as the NBRC hospital. The NBRC hospital differs greatly from the hospital you rotated through as a student.

For example, in the NBRC hospital the respiratory therapist can intubate, remove or reinsert a tracheostomy tube, perform needle decompression, and order CT-scans, chest X-rays and arterial blood gases. Limitations to what the respiratory therapist can do in the NBRC hospital are practically non-existent.

So, avoid making the mistake of answering exam questions based on what you could do during your non-NBRC clinical rotations.

The experienced staff therapist you followed as a student may be a truly wonderful therapist. However, it's possible that your clinical preceptor would get thrown out of the NBRC hospital.

Prioritizing Therapy

Many of the RRT exam questions ask what the therapist should do <u>FIRST</u>, or what the therapist should recommend <u>NEXT</u>? This is evident in both the free *and* paid NBRC practice exams. This is most likely because the NBRC wants to know if you can correctly prioritize the therapy you provide to your patients. A large part of being an effective and successful therapist involves knowing how to prioritize patient interventions.

A useful acronym to help you prioritize the therapy you recommend is **AVOC**. This stands for **Airway, Ventilation, Oxygenation, and Circulation**.

If you've recently taken BLS or ACLS, this may be confusing. These American Heart Association's courses now teach circulation as the first priority. However, in the NBRC hospital, we will first open the airway and then provide ventilation, oxygenation, and support of circulation.

These priorities represent the correct order therapy should be given to successfully pass the RRT exam. When you encounter a test question asking what the therapist should recommend first or what the therapist should do next, think of the following list.

Order of importance in the NBRC hospital
1. Airway
2. Ventilation
3. Oxygenation
4. Circulation/Perfusion

Check out the following example questions to practice your skills at prioritization.

Example 1: A patient receiving mechanical ventilation becomes cyanotic. The respiratory therapist determines the tracheostomy tube is dislodged. What should the therapist do <u>FIRST</u>; remove and replace the tracheostomy tube, increase the set respiratory rate, or increase the Fio2?
Answer: You must remove and replace the airway before you can ventilate and oxygenate the patient.

Example 2: A patient is placed on CPAP in an attempt to wean them from mechanical ventilation. The patient becomes apneic *and* hypoxemic. What should the respiratory therapist do FIRST; increase the Fio2 or provide ventilation?
Answer: Giving oxygen is of no help if the patient is not breathing. Treat the apnea, because ventilation is a priority over oxygenation.

Example 3: A patient is hypoxemic and bradycardic. What should the respiratory therapist do <u>FIRST</u>; give oxygen or Atropine?
Answer: Give oxygen first, because in the NBRC hospital, oxygenation is still a priority over circulation.

Choosing The Best Answer

Sometimes, all four answers appear to be correct. This is a tricky method the NBRC uses to further test your skills at prioritization. For this type of question, <u>the correct answer is again the one the therapist should do first.</u> Check out the following examples.

Question 1

What should the respiratory therapist recommend for a febrile patient admitted with pneumonia?

    A. Incentive Spirometry
    B. Chest physiotherapy
    C. Antibiotics
    D. Deep breathing and coughing maneuvers

As you can see, these are all excellent choices for a patient with pneumonia. However, <u>the correct answer is antibiotics</u> because treating the infection should be performed first.

Question 2

What should the respiratory therapist recommend for a febrile patient admitted with pneumonia and a Spo2 of 85% on room air.

    A. Incentive spirometry
    B. Chest physiotherapy
    C. Antibiotics
    D. Oxygen therapy

Again, these are all appropriate treatments for a patient with pneumonia. However, the information in the question changed. This time, the patient's Spo2 was 85%. Here, <u>the correct answer is oxygen therapy.</u> Supporting the patient's need for oxygen takes priority over fighting the infection with antibiotics.

Treating Stable vs. Unstable Patients

The stability of the patient is an important factor when deciding what to do first. For example, patients with a suspected pneumothorax will be treated differently depending upon how stable they are.

An unstable patient may need an immediate life saving intervention. A stable patient may have time for further diagnostic testing before a treatment is recommended.

Check out the following two similar test questions that require different answers depending on the stability of the patient.

Question 1

A hypotensive and tachycardic patient is suspected of having a pneumothorax. What should the therapist recommend <u>FIRST</u>?

    A. Portable chest X-ray
    B. Chest tube
    C. Needle decompression
    D. Arterial blood gas

Answer: A patient with hypotension and tachycardia is considered hemodynamically unstable. This patient requires an immediate intervention. Care of the patient should not be delayed.

    A. Incorrect. A portable chest X-ray would confirm the diagnosis, but takes too long for a hemodynamically unstable patient, who needs an <u>immediate intervention</u>.
    B. Incorrect. A chest tube will be needed, eventually, but takes too long to perform in a hemodynamically unstable patient, who needs an immediate intervention.
    C. Correct. The patient is hemodynamically **<u>unstable</u>** and needs an immediate intervention.
    D. Incorrect. An ABG will neither confirm the presence of a pneumothorax nor treat one.

Question 2

A patient receiving mechanical ventilation is suspected of having a pneumothorax due to diminished breath sounds on the right side and increased peak airway pressures. Vital sign reveal HR 98, RR 24, Bp 120/80. What should the therapist recommend FIRST?

    A. Portable chest X-ray
    B. Chest tube

C. Needle decompression
D. Arterial blood gas

Answer: This patient is also suspected of having a pneumothorax. However, the patient's vital signs are stable. As a result, this patient does not require an immediate intervention. Treatment of the pneumothorax can wait until it is confirmed with a chest X-ray.

A. Correct. The correct answer, this time is portable chest X-ray. This patient is hemodynamically stable. Therefore, the respiratory therapist has time to confirm the presence of a pneumothorax with a portable chest X-ray.

B. Incorrect. Because the patient is **stable**, there is time to confirm the presence of a pneumothorax with a chest X-ray.

C. Incorrect. Because the patient is stable, there is time to confirm the presence of a pneumothorax with a chest X-ray.

D. Incorrect. An ABG will neither confirm the presence of a pneumothorax nor treat one.

Physical Exam

Physical exam involves observing, palpating, percussing, and auscultating the patient. All of these methods reveal clues to the source of the patient's problems. Physical exam clues are included in a majority of questions on the respiratory therapy board exams.

Examination of the head and neck

Pursed lip breathing is a breathing technique used by COPD patients to control their shortness of breath.

Sternocleidomastoid muscles are located in the anterior part of the neck. These muscles may appear enlarged in-patients with COPD.

Nasal flaring is a sign of respiratory distress most often observed in children and infants.

Cyanosis

Cyanosis of the lips and/or mucous membranes is a severe sign of hypoxemia. **Recommend** oxygen for patients that are cyanotic.

Jugular Venous Distention (JVD)

Visual examination of the neck may reveal Jugular venous distension (JVD). JVD appears as a visible bulging of the external jugular veins in the neck. These jugular veins return blood from the head to the heart.

When the right side of the heart cannot pump blood fast enough due to right heart failure or volume overload, the jugular veins become distended.

Cor pulmonale (right heart failure), CHF (left heart failure), and chronic hypoxemia, due to COPD, are the most common causes of JVD. Simply put, patients with JVD may have heart failure, COPD, or both.

Tracheal Deviation

Tracheal deviation may be observed in some patients, using only a visual inspection. Palpation of the trachea may help confirm tracheal deviation and may also reveal subcutaneous emphysema. Subcutaneous emphysema is associated with barotrauma and pneumothorax, and may also result from dislodgement of the tracheostomy tube.

Palpation of the neck and conditions associated with tracheal deviation are covered in great detail later in this book.

Examination of the extremities and skin

Examination of the extremities and skin provides clues regarding the patient's circulation and perfusion.

Clubbing

Clubbing is an enlargement of the fingertips with an increased angle of the nail bed.

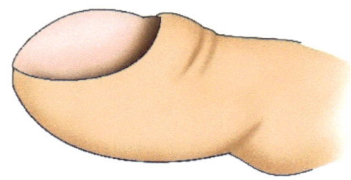

Chronic hypoxemia, due to lung and/or heart disease, is the most common cause of clubbing.

Recommend pulse-oximetry for patients with clubbing. Provide oxygen If the pulse-oximetry reading is low. However, be careful not to give too much oxygen to patients with COPD.

Recommend ECG and echocardiography if heart disease is suspected as a cause of clubbing.

Diaphoresis

Diaphoresis is unusually profuse sweating and is often a sign of an acute disease process, such as CHF or an infection. When a patient is diaphoretic look for other clues to determine its cause. Diaphoresis is associated with the following:

1. **Congestive Heart Failure (CHF).** CHF is also known as left sided heart failure.
   a. CHF may be associated with diaphoresis when other signs of potential heart failure, such as cardiomegaly, peripheral/pedal edema, and fine crackles during auscultation, are present.
   b. If CHF is suspected, **recommend** oxygen, positive inotropic agents to increase the strength of heart muscle contractions. Diuretics, such as Lasix (Furosemide), may also be recommended to remove excess fluid.
2. **Fever** is a common cause of diaphoresis.
   a. Fever may be associated with diaphoresis if the patient also has signs of infection such as a productive cough with yellow sputum.
   b. Treatment for bacterial infection includes antibiotics.
3. **Tuberculosis** is a less common cause of diaphoresis. An acid-fast bacillus (AFB) test of the patient's sputum is used to confirm an active tuberculosis infection.
   a. Tuberculosis may be associated with diaphoresis if it occurs at night or is described as night sweats. Tuberculosis is confirmed using an AFB (acid-fast bacillus) test of the sputum.
   b. **Recommend** anti-tuberculin drugs, such as Streptomycin or Rifampicin.
4. **Anxiety** may also cause diaphoresis.
   a. Anxiety may be associated with diaphoresis if the patient is nervous, apprehensive, or feels stressed.
   b. **Recommendations may include** sedatives, such as Lorazepam (Ativan).

Practice Question 1

A patient is diaphoretic with an axillary temperature of 102 F. The most appropriate treatment is?

  A. Diuretics
  B. Positive inotropic agents
  C. Antibiotics
  D. Morphine

Answer

  A. Incorrect. There is no evidence of heart failure or fluid overload as a cause of the diaphoresis.
  B. Incorrect. There is no information leading us to suspect CHF.
  C. Correct. The patient's diaphoresis and fever indicate a possibility of infection. Therefore, antibiotics are the correct response.
  D. Incorrect. Morphine

Practice Question 2

A patient is diaphoretic *and* hypoxemic with an axillary temperature of 102 F. The most appropriate treatment is:

  A. Diuretics
  B. Oxygen
  C. Antibiotics
  D. Positive inotropic agents

Answer

  A. Incorrect. The patient is diaphoretic; however, there is no sign of congestive heart failure.
  B. Correct. This is similar to question 1; however, now the patient is hypoxemic.
  C. Incorrect. Antibiotics are indicated; however, the priority here is oxygenation. Therefore, oxygen is the most appropriate treatment.
  D. Incorrect. There is no evidence of heart failure.

Practice Question 3

A patient with peripheral edema, diaphoresis and a Spo2 of 87% presents to the emergency room. What should the therapist recommend first?

    A. Oxygen
    B. Diuretics
    C. Positive inotropic agents
    D. Antibiotics

Answer

    A. Correct. In this question oxygen is again the priority. This is due to the Spo2 of 87% indicating hypoxemia.
    B. Incorrect. Diuretics may be needed but is not the first priority in a hypoxemic patient.
    C. Incorrect. Positive inotropic agents may be needed but are not the first priority in a hypoxemic patient.
    D. Incorrect. Antibiotics could be recommended if the patient had a fever or other sign of bacterial infection. There is no indication the patient has a bacterial infection.

Skin color

Abnormal skin color may appear cyanotic, jaundiced, pale, or ashen. Erythema is also abnormal. These all can be serious signs that point you in very specific directions in terms of how to answer the test question.

1. **Cyanosis** appears as blue or dusky skin and is due to hypoxemia. There are two primary types of cyanosis:

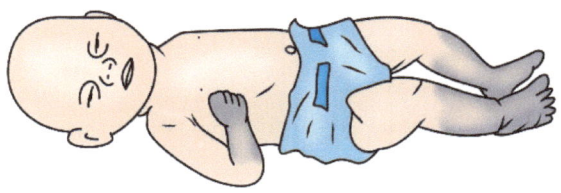

    a. Peripheral Cyanosis is often used interchangeably with the term acrocyanosis. This is a bluish discoloration of the digits and limbs due to circulatory insufficiency or failure. Peripheral cyanosis/acrocyanosis is not a sign of hypoxemia. Therefore, by itself, it does not require oxygen.

b. <u>Central Cyanosis</u> – is a bluish discoloration of the lips and oral mucosa and is a sign of hypoxemia. Central cyanosis is a true cyanosis and needs to be treated with oxygen first.

2. **Jaundice** is a yellow discoloration of the skin due to elevated bilirubin levels.

a. Jaundice is associated with liver failure and may also be associated with ascites. Ascites appears as a distended abdomen.

3. **Erythema** is a red, irritated, or burned part of the skin. Erythema is associated with:

a. Burns – Transcutaneous electrodes provide continuous non-invasive monitoring of oxygen and carbon dioxide in the capillaries and tissue underneath the probe. They function by heating the skin to cause capillary dilation. Unfortunately, transcutaneous electrodes are also a frequent cause of erythema, due to their use of heat. If the position of the electrode is not changed every 2 to 4 hours erythema may develop. If a test question notes erythema has developed around the site of a transcutaneous electrode, <u>the electrode must be removed</u>.

b. Infection – localized infections may cause erythema of the skin. **Recommend antibiotics.**

4. **Pale or ashen** skin color may indicate hypoxemia and/or anemia. **Recommend oxygen.**

Skin Temperature

Normal skin temperature ranges from 97 and 99.5 degrees Fahrenheit and 36.5 to 37.5 degree Celsius.

a. Cold peripheral skin temperature occurs in patients with heart failure and shock, due to the shunting of blood to the bodies' vital organs.

b. Warm or hot peripheral skin temperature occurs in patients with fever due to infection. **Recommend** supplemental oxygen if signs of hypoxemia exist and antibiotics.

Capillary Refill Time

The time it takes for color to return to normal when the nail bed is blanched is known as capillary refill time. Capillary refill time reflects the status of the patient's circulatory system and peripheral perfusion. Therefore, it is often used to determine the presence of shock and dehydration.

Technique: Press the patient's fingernail until it blanches. Release the fingernail and count the number of seconds it takes to return to normal color. Normal capillary refill time is less than 3 seconds.

Poor capillary refill is associated with poor cardiac output and poor perfusion to the extremities. In these patients color will take longer to return when the nail bed is pressed. Conditions such as shock, dehydration, and peripheral vascular disease are associated with poor capillary refill time.

Edema

Edema appears as swelling due to an abnormal accumulation of excess fluid. **Peripheral edema** affects the extremities. **Pedal edema** affects the ankles and feet. The ankles are most often affected due to the effect of gravity. Peripheral edema is measured by pressing on the site of the edema with the fingertips. This pressure causes pitting where the skin is pressed. The pitting is then rated on a scale of 1 to 4. Level 1 represents only slight edema, while level 4 represents severe edema.

Peripheral and pedal edema are associated with fluid overload, congestive heart failure (CHF), and renal failure.

Treatment may include diuretics and/or positive inotropic agents. Lasix (Furosemide) is a commonly recommended diuretic.

Ascites

Ascites is a form of edema that occurs in the abdomen. Ascites is most often associated with liver diseases such as cirrhosis. Ascites is less commonly associated with cancer and appendicitis. The hallmark sign of ascites is a distended abdomen that is dull to percussion.

Skin Turgor

Skin turgor can be used to assess a patient's hydration level. To perform the test, skin on the back of the hand or arm is gently pinched and pulled. A hydrated patient's skin will quickly return to its original configuration. A dehydrated patient's skin will return to its original configuration slowly and may remain raised for some time.

Practice Question 4
A patient presents to the emergency room with acute onset of shortness of breath. The patient is diaphoretic and has fine crackles in the lung bases. The patient's temperature is 98.8. The patient most likely has:
  A. Pneumonia
  B. Pneumothorax
  C. Congestive heart failure
  D. Pleural effusion

Answer
  A. Incorrect. A patient with pneumonia would more likely have coarse crackles. The sweating could result from a bacterial pneumonia in a patient with fever; however, this patient has a normal temperature.
  B. Incorrect. Lung sounds would be diminished in the location of a pneumothorax.
  C. Correct. Profuse sweating, also known as diaphoresis, is common in a patient with CHF. Diaphoresis can be caused by fever; however, the patient's temperature is normal. The fine crackles noted in the patient's lung bases are also consistent with CHF.

D. Incorrect. Pleural effusion does not cause diaphoresis and is not a cause of acute onset shortness of breath.

Chest Inspection

Respiratory pattern

Respiratory pattern is often used as one of several clues in the test question. Sometimes, the pattern helps you piece together the overall picture of what is happening with the patient. Other times, the respiratory pattern may clearly lead you to the answer. For example, a patient with Biot's, Cheyne-stokes, or an apneustic respiratory pattern should lead you to consider CNS pathologies, such as stroke or trauma to the brain. The patient's respiratory pattern provides excellent clues as to what disease process the test question may be leading you towards.

Eupnea is <u>normal</u> breathing.

Apnea is the <u>absence</u> of breathing.

Bradypnea is a <u>slow rate</u> of breathing, less than 12 breaths/min.

Hypopnea is <u>shallow</u> breathing.

Hyperpnea is <u>deep</u> breathing.

Tachypnea is <u>fast rate</u> of breathing.

Kussmaul's is <u>fast and deep</u> breathing. Kussmaul's respiratory pattern is associated with metabolic acidosis and diabetic ketoacidosis.

Biot's is <u>also fast and deep</u> with a pause at peak inspiration and an irregular exhalation. The rate is also irregular with periods of <u>apnea</u>. Biot's is associated with stroke and other CNS pathologies.

Cheyne-stokes respirations gradually increase in rate and depth and then gradually decrease in rate and depth. A period of apnea follows and then the cycle restarts. Cheyne-stokes respirations are associated with heart failure and stroke.

Apneustic is <u>prolonged gasping inhalations</u>. Associated with stroke, brain damage, brain tumors, and traumas.

<u>Practice Question 5</u>

A patient with a history of diabetes is breathing fast and deep. The patient's respiratory pattern is most likely?

- A. Biot's
- B. Tachypnea
- C. Kussmaul's
- D. Hyperpnea

Answer

- A. Incorrect. Biot's respiratory pattern is fast and deep but not associated with diabetes.
- B. Incorrect. Tachypnea is a fast rate of breathing.
- C. Correct. Kussmaul's respiratory pattern is fast and deep breathing and is associated with diabetic ketoacidosis.
- D. Incorrect. Hyperpnea is deep breathing.

Work of breathing

Normal Work of Breathing
Patients with a normal work of breathing have a normal respiratory rate and rhythm. The abdomen moves gently outward with inhalation and inward with exhalation. The accessory muscles of respiration are only slightly active.

Labored or Increased Work of Breathing
Signs of labored breathing include increased accessory muscle use, retractions, tracheal tugging, nasal flaring, and the patient's subjective complaint of shortness of breath and/or dyspnea.

1. **Accessory muscle use** is associated with increased airway resistance and muscle fatigue. Accessory muscles include the scalene, sternocleidomastoid, pectoralis major, trapezius, and internal intercostal.
2. **Retractions** appear as an inward depression of the skin around the chest wall, caused by forceful inspiration. Retractions may appear in the intercostal, supraclavicular, and sternal regions. Retractions are a sign of severe airway obstruction and/or respiratory distress.
3. **Tracheal tugging** occurs when the trachea moves downward during inspiration. This is due to the

generation of large negative pressures to overcome airway resistance.
4. **Nasal flaring** is a common sign of increased work of breathing in children and infants.

Practice Question 6
An adult patient in the ICU is breathing 22 breaths per minute with slightly active accessory muscles of respiration. This respiratory pattern could best be described as?
  A. Apneustic
  B. Hypopnea
  C. Tachypnea
  D. Eupnea

Answer
  A. Incorrect. Apneustic breathing appears as prolonged gasping inhalations.
  B. Incorrect. Hypopnea appears as shallow breathing.
  C. Incorrect. Tachypnea is a fast rate of breathing equal to more than 30 breaths per minute.
  D. Correct. This normal respiratory pattern is known as eupnea. Normal respiratory rate is less than 30 breaths per minute. Slightly active accessory muscles of respiration are also considered normal.

Practice Question 7
Increased accessory muscle use is most often due to?
  A. Hyperventilation
  B. Increased airway resistance
  C. Increased lung compliance
  D. Poor cardiac output

Answer
  A. Incorrect. Patients can hyperventilate without increasing their accessory muscle use.
  B. Correct. Increased airway resistance is the most common cause of increased accessory muscle use.

C. Incorrect. Increased lung compliance does not increase accessory muscle use. Decreased lung compliance may increase accessory muscle use.
D. Incorrect. Cardiac output does not affect accessory muscle use.

Thoracic configuration

Normal configuration– The chest diameter from front to back should be less than the side-to-side diameter. In more technical terms, the Anterior-posterior diameter should be less than the transverse diameter.

Abnormal configurations

1. **Atrophy** – Both neuromuscular disease and prolonged mechanical ventilation can cause wasting away of the accessory muscles. These patients often have trouble clearing airway secretions. The respiratory therapist can **recommend** the patient use an in-exsufflation device to assist with airway secretion clearance.

2. **Hypertrophy** – Patients with severe COPD rely on their accessory muscles of respiration to breath, even while at rest. This is due to the loss of elastic recoil in their lungs and displacement of the diaphragm, due to air trapping. As a result, the accessory muscles of respiration become enlarged.

3. **Barrel chest** – Patients with severe COPD may have increased A-P diameter due to hypertrophy of accessory muscles and hyperinflation (air trapping). Think of the terminology barrel chest, air trapping, increased A-P diameter, and hyperinflation as all being synonymous and also associated with COPD.

Restrictive thoracic configurations prevent full chest expansion. Ventilation is adversely affected as a result.

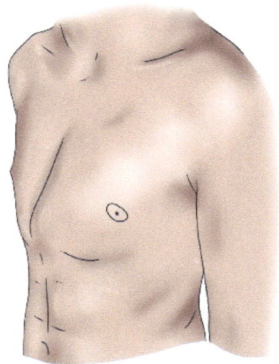

1. **Pectus carinatum** is an outward protrusion of the sternum. Often, this is referred to as pigeon chest. If severe enough, pectus carinatum will cause a restrictive lung defect. Recommend pulmonary function testing to determine the degree of restriction.

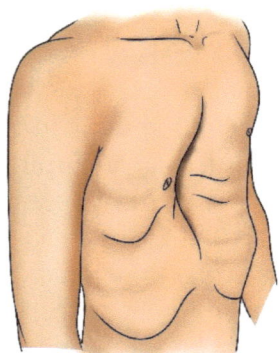

2. **Pectus excavatum** is a depressed sternum. If severe enough, pectus excavatum will cause a restrictive lung defect. Recommend pulmonary function testing to determine the degree of restriction.

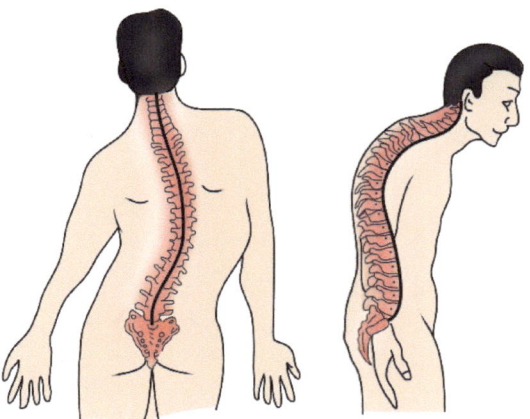

3. **Scoliosis** is a <u>lateral</u> curvature of the spine that results in restrictive lung disease.
4. **Kyphosis** is a <u>forward</u> curvature of the spine that causes the patient to lean forward. Kyphosis causes a restrictive lung defect.
5. **Kyphoscoliosis** is a <u>combination of both</u> a forward and a lateral curvature of the spine. Kyphoscoliosis causes a restrictive lung defect.

Palpation of the Chest

Palpation of the chest involves measuring chest expansion for symmetry, percussing the chest, and palpating for tactile fremitus.

Chest expansion

Evaluate chest expansion by placing both hands on the patient's chest and measuring the distance each hand moves apart during inhalation. Symmetrical chest expansion on both sides is normal.

Asymmetrical or unilateral chest movement is abnormal. Asymmetrical chest movement is associated with:

1. Pneumothorax
2. Atelectasis
3. Right mainstem intubation
4. Lobar consolidation
5. Lung resection
6. **Flail chest** is caused by <u>severe chest wall trauma,</u> such as multiple broken ribs. Flail chest causes paradoxical motion of the affected side as compared to the normal side of the chest.
7. **Seesaw movement** of the abdomen and chest occurs when the diaphragm fatigues, as observed in paralyzed patients. This should not be confused with flail chest.

Decreased chest expansion is associated with:

1. Neuromuscular diseases such as Myasthenia Gravis or Guillain-Barre syndrome. Other neuromuscular diseases causing decreased chest expansion may include stroke, Parkinson's disease, and amyotrophic lateral sclerosis (ALS).
2. COPD may also cause decreased chest expansion due to pre-existing hyperinflation of the chest.

Chest Percussion (Diagnostic)

Percussing the chest wall produces distinct sounds that help evaluate the underlying tissue. Percussing the chest can aid in the diagnosis of pneumothorax, pneumonia, pleural effusion, COPD and many other disease processes.

Technique:

1. First, place only the middle finger firmly against the chest and between the ribs. Strike the first joint of the middle finger with your opposite middle finger tip.
2. Next, evaluate the intensity (loudness) and pitch, while comparing both sides of the chest.

Normal chest percussion

A normal lung should produce an easily heard low-pitched sound when percussed. This is known as resonant.

Abnormal chest percussion

1. **Dull or decreased resonance** occurs when the density in or around the lung increases. Causes of dull or decreased resonance include:
    a. Pleural effusion
    b. Pneumonia
    c. Atelectasis
    d. Lung tumors
2. **Hyperresonant** – A hyperresonant lung produces a loud, hollow sound. Both pneumothorax and COPD are hyperresonant, due to excessive air trapped in the lung or pleural space.
3. **Tympanic** – The stomach normally produces a tympanic sound when percussed. Tympany is a drum like sound. A lung that is tympanic to percussion may indicate air trapping or pneumothorax.

Practice Question 8

A patient with multiple right-sided rib fractures would present with which of the following findings?
   A. Dull percussion on right side
   B. See-saw chest movement

C. Symmetrical chest expansion
D. Flail chest

Answer
A. Incorrect. Percussion is not assessed on a patient with broken ribs. In addition, percussion may or may not be affected, depending on if the lung is affected or there is excessive bleeding.
B. Incorrect. Seesaw chest movement is a sign of diaphragm fatigue, rather than chest trauma.
C. Incorrect. Chest expansion would be asymmetrical in a patient with broken ribs.
D. Correct. Flail chest is associated with severe chest wall trauma.

Tactile Fremitus

Fremitus is another word for vibrations. Vibrations from the patient's speech are known as vocal fremitus. Vibrations felt by the clinician's hands when they are placed on the patient's chest are known as tactile fremitus. The clinician describes the vibrations as increased, decreased, or absent.

Vibrations are transmitted better through consolidated lungs than clear lungs. However, it is important to note this does not apply to pleural effusions. Because pleural effusions occur outside the lung, they lack any connection with an airway. As a result, pleural effusions do not transmit voice sounds well. Thus, tactile fremitus is decreased over a pleural effusion.

Technique:

1. Have the patient repeat the word "ninety-nine" while palpating the anterior, posterior, and lateral chest wall with your fingertips.
2. Note if the vibrations (fremitus) are increased, decreased, or absent.

Increased fremitus is associated with:

1. Pneumonia
2. Lung tumors

3. Atelectasis

Decreased fremitus is associated with:

1. COPD
2. Pneumothorax
3. Pleural effusions
4. Obese or very muscular patients

Rhoncial fremitus is associated with secretions and can usually be cleared with a cough.

Crepitus

Subcutaneous emphysema (air under the skin) is a common cause of crepitus. Crepitus feels like crackling under the skin when palpating the neck, jaw, and clavicles. Crepitus often results from barotrauma, due to vigorous bagging and/or mechanical ventilation.

Tracheal Palpation

Understanding which direction the trachea shifts in patients with pneumonia, pleural effusion, pneumothorax, or atelectasis will greatly increase your chances of passing the board exams.

Use these two simple facts to help you decide what could be causing the tracheal shift.

1. Lung problems outside the lung, such as pleural effusions or pneumothorax, push the trachea away
2. Lung problems inside the lung, such as pneumonia or atelectasis, pull the trachea towards them.

Practice Question 9
Increased tactile fremitus is noted in the patient's right lower lobe. Which of the following conditions would explain this?
   A. Pneumothorax
   B. Pneumonia
   C. Pleural effusion
   D. COPD

Answer

A. Incorrect. Pneumothorax is associated with decreased fremitus, due to excessive air in the pleural space.
B. Correct. Consolidations, such as pneumonia, transmit vibrations well.
C. Incorrect. Pleural effusions lack an attached or conducting airway to transmit vibrations.
D. Incorrect. COPD is associated with decreased fremitus due to air trapping.

Practice Question 10
Palpation of the patient's trachea reveals a tracheal shift to the right side. Which of the following would most likely cause this finding?
A. Right side atelectasis
B. Right side pneumothorax
C. Right side pleural effusion
D. Left side pneumonia

Answer
A. Correct. Lung problems inside the lung pull the trachea toward them.
B. Incorrect. Lung problems outside the lung push the trachea away.
C. Incorrect. Lung problems outside the lung push the trachea away.
D. Incorrect. Lung problems inside the lung pull the trachea toward them.

Tenderness

Tenderness in regions of the chest may be due to surgical procedures or other traumas. Avoid areas of tenderness during chest inspection.

Do not recommend manual chest percussion to patients who have just undergone thoracic surgery, as this is a relative contraindication.

Do Recommend Deep breathing and vibratory PEP therapy for patient's who have undergone thoracic surgery.

Auscultation of the lungs

Breath sound Characteristics

1. Pitch may be low, moderate, or high
2. Intensity may be soft, moderate, or loud
3. Duration may be continuous or discontinuous
4. Inspiratory vs. expiratory

Normal breath sounds

Vesicular, bronchial, and bronchovesicular breath sounds are considered normal when heard in specific regions of the lung.

1. **Vesicular** breath sounds are quiet, low pitched, soft intensity sounds heard over the peripheral (outer) lung regions.
2. **Bronchial** breath sounds are harsh, loud sounds. Bronchial breath sounds are heard over the large airways, such as the bronchial tubes and trachea. Bronchial breath sounds heard over the lung bases would suggest a consolidation, such as pneumonia.
3. **Bronchovesicular** is a combination of bronchial and vesicular breath sounds. Bronchovesicular breath sounds are normal when heard over the sternum and upper scapulae.

Abnormal Breath Sounds

Bronchial breath sounds heard over the peripheral regions of the lung, and diminished breath sounds are abnormal. Technically, these breath sounds are not considered adventitious, because they are not added sounds superimposed on top of normal sounds.

1. **Abnormal bronchial** breath sounds replace vesicular sounds when that part of the lung increases in density. Pneumonia may cause bronchial breath sounds, where vesicular breath sounds should be heard. If a test question states bronchial breath sounds are heard in the

lung bases or periphery, you should <u>suspect a consolidation, such as pneumonia</u>.

2. **Diminished breath sounds** may sometimes be referred to as distant on the NBRC exam. Anything that causes a reduction of airflow or blocks the transmission of sound through the lung may cause diminished breath sounds. Here are examples:

   a. <u>Pneumothorax</u> causes air to accumulate in the pleural space and reduces air movement in the collapsed lung. Diminished or distant breath sounds may indicate pneumothorax. However, **absent breath sounds** are a hallmark sign of pneumothorax.

   b. <u>Pleural effusions</u> cause fluid to accumulate in the pleural space. This creates a physical barrier to transmission of breath sounds.

   c. <u>COPD</u> patients have diminished breath sounds, due to air trapping and hyperinflated lungs.

   d. <u>Foreign body airway obstruction</u> and <u>mucous plugging</u> may also reduce airflow, causing diminished breath sounds over the obstructed lung.

   e. <u>Obese patients</u> may have diminished breath sounds, due to poor sound transmission.

   f. <u>Overly sedated patients</u> may have diminished breath sounds, due to shallow or slow breathing.

Adventitious breath sounds

Adventitious breath sounds are abnormal added or extra sounds superimposed over normal breath sounds during auscultation of the lungs.

1. **Wheeze** is a continuous high-pitched sound. Wheezing may be polyphonic or monophonic. Polyphonic wheezing is associated with narrowing of multiple bronchial tubes. Monophonic wheezing is associated with only one narrowed bronchial tube. Wheezing may be caused by:

a. **Asthma** – If due to asthma <u>wheezing should be bilateral</u>. There is no such thing as unilateral asthma. Recommend aerosolized albuterol if wheezing is bilateral and asthma is suspected. If breath sounds change from wheezing to markedly diminished after receiving aerosolized albuterol, the patient is getting worse and needs more aggressive therapy. Recommend a continuous nebulizer with a higher dose of albuterol.

b. **Foreign body airway obstruction** – Unilateral wheezing is highly suspicious for foreign body airway obstruction, particularly in a child. **<u>Aspirated foreign bodies such as plastics are radiopaque. As a result, chest X-ray cannot be used to rule out a foreign body airway obstruction.</u>** Unilateral wheezing caused by foreign body aspiration can be treated with rigid bronchoscopy. If the patient shows signs of hypoxemia you must remember your priorities and <u>give oxygen first.</u>

2. **Fine crackles** are most often due to pulmonary edema and atelectasis. <u>Fine crackles cannot be cleared with suctioning</u>. For patients with fine crackles, due to CHF/pulmonary edema, **recommend**:

   a. <u>Oxygen</u> if the patient has signs of hypoxemia, such as low Spo2 or increased heart rate.
   b. <u>CPAP/BiPAP</u> to apply positive airway pressure.
   c. <u>Positive inotropes,</u> such as digoxin, to increase the strength of the hearts contractions.
   d. <u>Diuretics,</u> such as Lasix and Furosemide.

For patients with fine crackles, due to atelectasis, recommend:

   a. <u>Oxygen</u> if the patient has signs of hypoxemia such as low Spo2 or increased heart rate.
   b. <u>Incentive spirometer.</u>

3. **Coarse crackles** occur when secretions move in the airways, due to pneumonia or bronchitis. Coarse crackles

due to secretions, are heard on both inhalation and exhalation. Recommend coughing and/or suctioning for patients with coarse crackles.

4. **Stridor** is a serious sign of airway obstruction. This can be due to foreign body airway obstruction, post extubation edema, or croup. Stridor is audible mostly during inspiration. Treatment of stridor depends on its severity:

    a. **Mild/moderate stridor** – If stridor is only moderate and the patient is not unstable, you will have time to treat it without intubation. **Recommend:**
        - Oxygen and racemic epinephrine for a stable patient with mild or moderate stridor.
        - Suctioning if secretions are suspected of causing mild or moderate stridor. Be careful with recommending suctioning for patients with stridor. The patient must be stable and have only mild or moderate stridor to recommend suctioning.
        - Rigid bronchoscopy if foreign body airway obstruction is suspected.

    b. **Severe stridor** – Severe stridor often occurs in patients with epiglottitis. Severe stridor compromises both ventilation and oxygenation of the patient. This is a dangerous situation for the patient. They will often have additional signs, indicating they are unstable. They may be cyanotic, have severe retractions, or be hypotensive. There is no time for recommending tests that will delay care of this patient. Severe stridor requires immediate intervention. Therefore, **recommend intubation** for a patient with severe stridor.

5. **Pleural friction rub** sounds like creaking or grating. It occurs when the visceral and parietal pleura are inflamed and rub together. Treatment for pleural friction rub includes steroids to reduce inflammation and antibiotics to treat infection.

Practice Question 11

Auscultation of a patient's lungs reveals coarse bilateral crackles. This is most likely due to?

    A. Secretions
    B. Pulmonary edema
    C. Pulmonary fibrosis
    D. Atelectasis

Answer

    A. Correct. Coarse crackles are associated with secretions.
    B. Incorrect. Pulmonary edema is associated with fine crackles.
    C. Incorrect. Pulmonary fibrosis is associated with fine crackles.
    D. Incorrect. Atelectasis is associated with fine crackles.

Practice Question 12

Auscultation of a 3-year-old child's lungs reveals unilateral wheezing and a strong non-productive cough. A portable chest X-ray performed in the ER is clear. This patient most likely has?

    A. Asthma
    B. Secretions in the airway
    C. Foreign body airway obstruction
    D. Pneumonia

Answer

    A. Incorrect. Asthma does not affect only one side of the lung.
    B. Incorrect. Secretions in the airway would produce coarse crackles when auscultated.
    C. Correct. Unilateral wheezing in a child is highly suspicious for foreign body airway obstruction. Aspirated foreign bodies, such as plastics, may be radiopaque. As a result, chest X-ray cannot rule out foreign body airway obstruction.
    D. Incorrect. Pneumonia would produce bronchial breath sounds when auscultated.

Practice Question 13

An unstable patient is noted to have signs and symptoms of a pneumothorax. What should the therapist recommend NEXT?
- A. Obtain an ABG
- B. Order a chest X-ray
- C. Needle decompression
- D. Chest tube insertion

Answer
- A. Incorrect. An arterial blood gas cannot confirm or rule out a pneumothorax.
- B. Incorrect. A chest X-ray could help confirm a pneumothorax; however, this unstable patient needs an immediate intervention. A chest X-ray takes too long to obtain and would delay care of this unstable patient.
- C. Correct. This patient is unstable and needs an immediate intervention. Needle decompression is the quickest and most appropriate intervention.
- D. Incorrect. Chest tube insertion will be needed; however, this takes too long and delays care to an unstable patient, needing an immediate intervention.

Auscultation of voice sounds

Auscultation of voice sounds helps detect lung consolidations such as pneumonia. Voice sounds change as they pass through consolidated lungs. Any change in voice sound or intensity while auscultating may indicate pneumonia.

1. **Egophony** – While auscultating each lung field, the patient is instructed to say the letter "E". In normal lungs, with no disease process, the E will sound like an E. However, when there is a consolidation, such as with pneumonia, the "E" will sound like an "A".
2. **Bronchophony** – While auscultating each lung field, the patient is instructed to recite the word "ninety-nine". If an increased intensity and clarity is noted, the patient may have a consolidation, such as pneumonia.
3. **Whispered pectoriloquy** – While auscultating each lung field, the patient is instructed to whisper "ninety-nine". If these words are clear it suggests a consolidation, such as pneumonia.

Auscultation of heart sounds

Normal heart sounds in the adult are known as S1 and S2. This represents the classic lub-dub sound the heart makes as it beats. The lub corresponds to S1 and the dub corresponds to S2. When there are added or extra sounds this is abnormal in the adult. An S3 or S4 sound, or a heart that makes a galloping sound is an indication to recommend an echocardiogram and ECG.

Abnormal heart sounds

1. **S3 and S4** are abnormal heart sounds that may indicate cardiac anomalies or heart failure. Remember, S3 is a normal heart sound in many children.
2. **Murmurs** are the abnormal sounds turbulent blood flow makes as it passes through the heart.
3. **Bruits** are the sounds turbulent blood flow makes as it passes through a blood vessel, such as the carotid artery.

4. **P2** is the sound the pulmonary valve makes when it closes. A loud P2 may indicate pulmonary hypertension.
5. **Gallop rhythm** may indicate heart failure.

Recommend an echocardiogram and ECG for any abnormal heart sounds.

Practice Question 14

While auscultating voice sounds the respiratory therapist instructs the patient to whisper the words "ninety-nine". The therapist can clearly hear the patient whisper "ninety-nine" while auscultating the right lower lobe. The patient most likely has?

    A. Right lower lobe pneumonia
    B. Asthma
    C. Normal lungs
    D. Right side pneumothorax

Answer

    A. Correct. Using the whispered pectoriloquy technique, if the whispered words are auscultated clearly, there is a consolidation present such as pneumonia.
    B. Incorrect. Asthma is associated with air trapping, which does not transmit sound well.
    C. Incorrect. Normal lungs would not transmit the whispered words well.
    D. Incorrect. Pneumothorax is associated with increased air in the pleural space. This would not transmit sound well.

Practice Question 15

While auscultating an adult patient's heart, the respiratory therapist notes a murmur. What should the therapist recommend NEXT?

    A. Oxygen
    B. Chest X-ray
    C. Echocardiogram
    D. CT-scan

Answer

A. Incorrect. There is no indication the patient needs oxygen.
B. Incorrect. Chest X-ray is not indicated for heart murmurs.
C. Correct. An echocardiogram can further assess heart function.
D. Incorrect. CT scan is not indicated for heart murmurs.

Pathology Quick Reference

Understand how physical exam of the patient relates to lung pathology.

Pneumothorax:
1. Absent breath sounds. Distant or diminished breath sounds are also used to describe pneumothorax.
2. Hyperresonant to percussion
3. Decreased fremitus, because vibrations travel poorly through the air.
4. Trachea shifts away from a pneumothorax, because a pneumothorax occurs outside the lung.

Pleural effusion:
1. Bronchial breath sounds
2. Dull percussion
3. Decreased fremitus, because pleural effusions are outside the lung where there is no conducting airway to transmit vibrations.
4. Trachea shifts away from a pleural effusion, because it occurs outside the lung.

Pneumonia
1. Bronchial breath sounds
2. Dull percussion
3. Increased fremitus
4. Trachea is pulled towards pneumonia because it is inside the lung.
5. Voice sounds are altered and increased in intensity

Asthma
1. Bilateral wheezing
2. Resonant to hyperresonant percussion on both sides due to air trapping.
3. Decreased or normal fremitus depending on the degree of air trapping.

Foreign body airway obstruction

1. Absent, distant, or diminished breath sounds unilaterally
2. Hyperresonant percussion on affected side, due to air trapping
3. Decreased or normal fremitus, depending on degree of air trapping.

Atelectasis

1. Fine crackles to auscultation
2. Dull percussion
3. Increased fremitus
4. Trachea is pulled towards the affected side if large amount of atelectasis.

Exam Practice Questions

These questions are not just questions; they are learning opportunities. They were developed, based on the newest and most up to date NBRC testing matrix.

1. Signs of pneumothorax include all of the following except?
   A. Absent breath sounds
   B. Dull percussion
   C. Decreased fremitus
   D. Hyper resonant percussion

2. While assessing a patient with a productive cough, the respiratory therapist notes the right upper lobe has increased tactile fremitus, is dull to percussion, and has bronchial breath sounds. The patient most likely has?
   A. Pleural effusion
   B. Pneumonia
   C. Pneumothorax
   D. Pulmonary edema

3. Increased accessory muscle use is most often due to?
   A. Increased airway resistance
   B. Increased lung compliance
   C. Pleural effusion
   D. Increased alveolar ventilation

4. While auscultating voice sounds, the therapist hears the soft A sound, or ahhhh, when the patient says the letter "E". This change in sound is associated with which of the following conditions?
   A. Pneumothorax
   B. Pneumonia
   C. Pulmonary Edema
   D. COPD

5. Vesicular lung sounds in the periphery of the lung fields may also be referred to as?

A. Rhonchi
B. Wheezing
C. Normal
D. Bronchial

6. Following endotracheal intubation, chest assessment reveals left sided breath sounds are absent and resonant to percussion. This is most likely due to?
A. Right mainstem intubation
B. Left side pneumothorax
C. Large pleural effusion
D. Previous left sided lobectomy

7. Assessment of a patient's left lung reveals absent breath sounds and hyperresonance to percussion. This is most likely due to?
A. Right mainstem intubation
B. Left side pneumothorax
C. Large pleural effusion
D. Pulmonary embolism

8. A patient receiving mechanical ventilation has distant breath sounds on the left side with a tracheal shift to the right. The therapist should suspect?
A. Right mainstem intubation
B. Left side pneumothorax
C. Left upper lobe pneumonia
D. Pulmonary embolus

9. The respiratory therapist is assessing a patient in the emergency room, who fell from a ladder while working outside. The chest X-ray has confirmed 5 broken ribs on the left side. Which of the following findings should the therapist expect to find while assessing the chest?
A. Symmetrical chest excursion
B. Flail chest
C. Increased fremitus on left side
D. See-saw movement of chest and abdomen

10. Coarse crackles auscultated bilaterally most likely indicate?
    A. Pulmonary edema
    B. Pulmonary fibrosis
    C. Airway secretions
    D. Atelectasis

11. A patient in the emergency room is noted to have substernal retractions, marked stridor, and central cyanosis. What should the respiratory therapist recommend at this time?
    A. Nebulized racemic epinephrine
    B. Intubation
    C. Beta 2 agonist
    D. Cool aerosol mask

12. The respiratory therapist assesses a patient receiving mechanical ventilation in the ICU. Left side breath sounds are distant during auscultation and hyperresonant to percussion. The right side is clear to auscultation and resonant to percussion. These findings most likely indicate?
    A. Right mainstem intubation
    B. Left pneumothorax
    C. Foreign body airway obstruction
    D. Unilateral Asthma

13. A patient with fine bilateral crackles most likely has which of the following?
    A. Pulmonary edema
    B. Pleural effusion
    C. Airway secretions
    D. Cystic fibrosis

14. A patient has just been extubated in the ICU. The respiratory therapist notes the patient has moderate stridor and intercostal retractions. The patient's heart rate is 98 beats per minute, their respiratory rate is 24,

and their blood pressure is 130/90. What should the
therapist recommend?
A. Racemic epinephrine
B. Re-intubation
C. Manual Bag-mask ventilation
D. Portable chest X-ray

15. Chest X-ray results confirm pneumonia in the right lower
    lobe of a patient. Auscultation of the right lower lobe
    would most likely reveal?
    A. Vesicular breath sounds
    B. Bronchial breath sounds
    C. Bronchovesicular breath sounds
    D. Stridor

16. A diaphoretic patient is found to have cardiomegaly on
    chest X-ray. Auscultation reveals fine crackles in the lung
    bases. This patient most likely has?
    A. Congestive Heart Failure
    B. Cor Pulmonale
    C. COPD
    D. Atelectasis

17. Which of the following signs may indicate a patient is
    dehydrated?
    A. Pedal edema
    B. Bilateral basal crackles
    C. Poor skin turgor
    D. Diaphoresis

18. Which of the following tests will best assess perfusion to
    a patient's extremities?

    A. Spo2
    B. Capillary refill
    C. Sweat test
    D. ABG

19. A patient with Kussmal's respiratory pattern most likely has which of the following pathologies?
    A. Diabetic ketoacidosis
    B. Ischemic Stroke
    C. Hemorrhagic stroke
    D. Brain trauma

20. Pneumothorax is suspected in a mechanically ventilated patient in the ICU. The patient is on assist control mode and has a size 8.0 ETT secured at 22cm at the lip. The patient is hemodynamically stable. What should the therapist recommend NEXT?
    A. Arterial blood gas
    B. Withdraw the ETT 2 cm
    C. Portable chest X-ray
    D. Switch to pressure control ventilation

Exam Practice Questions With Answers and Rationales

1. Signs of pneumothorax include all of the following except?
   A. Absent breath sounds
   B. Dull percussion
   C. Decreased fremitus
   D. Hyperresonant percussion

   Answer
   A. Incorrect. Absent breath sounds are a sign of pneumothorax.
   B. Correct. Dull percussion is not a sign of pneumothorax. Pneumothoraxes are hyperresonant to percussion due to air trapped in the pleural space.
   C. Incorrect. Decreased fremitus is a sign of pneumothorax, because sound travels poorly through air as compared to consolidations.
   D. Incorrect. Hyperresonance is a sign of pneumothorax.

2. While assessing a patient with a productive cough, the respiratory therapist notes the right upper lobe has increased tactile fremitus, is dull to percussion, and has bronchial breath sounds. The patient most likely has?
   A. Pleural effusion
   B. Pneumonia
   C. Pneumothorax
   D. Pulmonary edema

   Answer
   A. Incorrect. Pleural effusions have decreased fremitus because there is no connecting airway to the effusion to transmit sound vibrations.
   B. Correct. Pneumonia is associated with all of these signs.
   C. Incorrect. Pneumothorax includes none of these signs.

D. Incorrect. Pulmonary edema produces fine crackles, fremitus is normal, and percussion is resonant.

3. Increased accessory muscle use is most often due to?
   A. Increased airway resistance
   B. Increased lung compliance
   C. Pleural effusion
   D. Increased alveolar ventilation

   Answer
   A. **Correct.** Increased airway resistance imposes a greater workload on the patient's respiratory system. This increased workload often leads to an increase in accessory muscle use, particularly in patients with pre-existing pulmonary disease, such as COPD.
   B. Incorrect. Increased lung compliance does not increase the workload on the accessory muscles of respiration. Decreased lung compliance would increase the workload on the accessory muscles of respiration.
   C. Incorrect. A pleural effusion may not affect accessory muscle use.
   D. Incorrect. Alveolar ventilation may increase with no impact on accessory muscle use.

4. While auscultating voice sounds, the therapist hears the soft A sound, or ahhhh, when the patient says the letter "E". This change in sound is associated with which of the following conditions?
   A. Pneumothorax
   B. Pneumonia
   C. Pulmonary Edema
   D. COPD

   Answer
   A. Incorrect. Increased air does not alter voice sounds as they pass through the lungs.
   B. Correct. Pneumonia is a consolidation that alters sounds as it passes through.

C. Incorrect. Pulmonary edema is not a consolidation and does not alter sound as it passes through.

D. Incorrect. COPD is associated with air trapping. Air does not alter voice sounds as they pass through the lungs.

5. Vesicular lung sounds in the periphery of the lung fields may also be referred to as?
   A. Rhonchi
   B. Wheezing
   C. Normal
   D. Bronchial

   Answer
   A. Incorrect. Rhonchi are low-pitched discontinuous sounds that may be heard throughout the lungs.
   B. Incorrect. Wheezing are adventitious lung sounds that may be heard throughout the lungs.
   C. Correct. Vesicular sounds in the periphery of the lung fields are normal.
   D. Incorrect. Bronchial breath sounds are harsh, loud breath sounds auscultated over the large airways, such as the bronchial tubes and trachea.

6. Following endotracheal intubation, chest assessment reveals breath sounds on the left side are distant and resonant to percussion. This is most likely due to?
   A. Right mainstem intubation
   B. Left side pneumothorax
   C. Large pleural effusion
   D. Esophageal intubation

   Answer
   A. Correct. Distant breath sounds on the left side, following an intubation procedure is consistent with right mainstem intubation.
   B. Incorrect. Pneumothorax would reveal hyperresonance to percussion.

C. Incorrect. Pleural effusions would be dull to percussion.
D. Incorrect. There are no signs of esophageal intubation.

7. Assessment of a patient's left lung reveals absent breath sounds and hyperresonance to percussion. This is most likely due to?
A. Right mainstem intubation
B. Left side pneumothorax
C. Large pleural effusion
D. Pulmonary embolism

Answer
A. Incorrect. There is no information indicating this patient is intubated. In addition, the left lung would reveal normal or decreased resonance if there were a right mainstem intubation.
B. Correct. Left sided pneumothorax is associated with these findings.
C. Incorrect. A pleural effusion would reveal bronchial breath sounds and would be dull to percussion.
D. Incorrect. A pulmonary embolism does not affect breaths sounds or percussion.

8. A patient receiving mechanical ventilation has distant breath sounds on the left side with a tracheal shift to the right. The therapist should suspect?
A. Right mainstem intubation
B. Left side pneumothorax
C. Left upper lobe pneumonia
D. Pulmonary embolus

Answer
A. Incorrect. A right mainstem intubation would not shift the trachea.
B. Correct. Pneumothorax causes the trachea to shift away from it.

C. Incorrect. Unlike a pneumothorax, pneumonia occurs inside the lungs, therefore, the trachea is pulled towards the pneumonia.

D. Incorrect. Pulmonary embolus do not cause tracheal shift.

9. The respiratory therapist is assessing a patient in the emergency room, following a fall from a ladder. The chest X-ray has confirmed 5 broken ribs on the left side. Which of the following findings should the therapist expect to find while assessing the chest?
   A. Symmetrical chest excursion
   B. Flail chest
   C. Dull percussion
   D. See-saw movement of the chest and abdomen

Answer

A. Incorrect. Broken ribs will cause asymmetrical movement of the chest.

B. Correct. Flail chest causes paradoxical motion of the affected side as compared to the normal side of the chest.

C. Incorrect. Broken ribs should not be percussed.

D. Incorrect. Seesaw movement of the chest and abdomen is associated with diaphragmatic fatigue.

10. Coarse crackles auscultated bilaterally most likely indicate?
    A. Pulmonary edema
    B. Pulmonary fibrosis
    C. Airway secretions
    D. Atelectasis

Answer

A. Incorrect. Pulmonary edema is associated with fine crackles.

B. Incorrect. Pulmonary fibrosis is associated with fine crackles.

C. Correct. Airway secretions are associated with coarse crackles.

D. Incorrect. Atelectasis is associated with fine crackles.

11. A patient in the emergency room is noted to have substernal retractions, severe stridor, and central cyanosis. What should the respiratory therapist recommend at this time?
    A. Nebulized racemic epinephrine
    B. Intubation
    C. Beta 2 agonist
    D. Cool aerosol mask

    Answer
    A. Incorrect. This will delay care of an unstable patient, who requires immediate establishment of an airway.
    B. Correct. Immediate establishment of an airway is indicated in an unstable patient with severe stridor.
    C. Incorrect. Beta 2 agonist is not indicated for stridor.
    D. Incorrect. Cool aerosol mask will not treat severe stridor.

12. The respiratory therapist assesses a patient receiving mechanical ventilation in the ICU. Left side breath sounds are distant during auscultation and hyperresonant to percussion. The right side is clear to auscultation and resonant to percussion. These findings most likely indicate?
    A. Right mainstem intubation
    B. Left pneumothorax
    C. Foreign body airway obstruction
    D. Unilateral Asthma

    Answer
    A. Incorrect. Right mainstem intubation would not be associated with left side hyperresonance to percussion.

B. Correct. Distant or absent breath sounds and hyperresonance to percussion are associated with pneumothorax.
C. Incorrect. There is no information suggesting the patient inhaled a foreign body.
D. Incorrect. Unilateral asthma does not exist.

13. A patient with fine bilateral crackles most likely has?
   A. Pulmonary edema
   B. Pleural effusion
   C. Airway secretions
   D. Cystic fibrosis

Answer
   A. Correct. Fine bilateral crackles are associated with pulmonary edema.
   B. Incorrect. Pleural effusion is associated with bronchial breath sounds.
   C. Incorrect. Airway secretions are associated with coarse crackles.
   D. Incorrect. Cystic fibrosis is associated with airway secretions and coarse crackles.

14. A patient has just been extubated in the ICU. The respiratory therapist notes the patient has moderate stridor and mild intercostal retractions. What should the therapist recommend?
   A. Racemic epinephrine
   B. Re-intubation
   C. Manual Bag-mask ventilation
   D. Portable chest X-ray

Answer
   A. Correct. Racemic epinephrine is the best choice, as this will reduce glottis swelling post extubation in an otherwise stable patient.
   B. Incorrect. The patient only has moderate stridor, and there is no evidence in this question that the patient is unstable.

C. Incorrect. Manual ventilation is not a treatment for stridor.
D. Incorrect. Portable chest X-ray will neither treat nor identify subglottic swelling.

15. Chest X-ray results confirm pneumonia in the right lower lobe of a patient. Auscultation of the right lower lobe would most likely reveal?
A. Vesicular breath sounds
B. Bronchial breath sounds
C. Bronchovesicular breath sounds
D. Stridor

Answer
A. Incorrect. Vesicular breath sounds are quiet, low pitched, soft intensity sounds heard over the peripheral (outer) lung regions.
B. Correct. Bronchial breath sounds are associated with a consolidation such as pneumonia.
C. Incorrect. Bronchovesicular breath sounds are a combination of bronchial and vesicular breath sounds. Bronchovesicular breath sounds are normal when heard over the sternum and upper scapulae.
D. Incorrect. Stridor occurs in the upper airway.

16. A diaphoretic patient is found to have cardiomegaly on chest X-ray. Auscultation reveals fine crackles in the lung bases. This patient most likely has?
A. Congestive Heart Failure
B. Pneumonia
C. COPD
D. Atelectasis

Answer
A. Correct. Cardiomegaly, diaphoresis, and fine crackles are associated with congestive heart failure.
B. Incorrect. Neither fine crackles, nor cardiomegaly are associated with pneumonia.

C. Incorrect. COPD is not associated with diaphoresis and fine crackles in the lung bases.
D. Incorrect. Atelectasis is not associated with cardiomegaly and diaphoresis.

17. Which of the following signs may indicate a patient is dehydrated?
    A. Pedal edema
    B. Bilateral basal crackles
    C. Poor skin turgor
    D. Diaphoresis

    Answer
    A. Incorrect. Pedal edema is associated with fluid overload.
    B. Incorrect. Basal crackles are associated with fluid overload.
    C. Correct. Poor skin turgor is associated with dehydration.
    D. Incorrect. Diaphoresis is associated with fluid overload.

18. Which of the following tests will best assess perfusion to a patient's extremities?
    A. Spo2
    B. Capillary refill
    C. Sweat test
    D. ABG

    Answer
    A. Incorrect. The Spo2 reading from a pulse oximeter can give an inaccurate reading in the setting of poor perfusion; however, capillary refill is the best answer.
    B. Correct. Capillary refill provides a good assessment of perfusion to the extremities.
    C. Incorrect. A sweat test is not related to perfusion of the extremities.
    D. Incorrect. An ABG does not reflect perfusion of the extremities.

19. A patient with Kussmaul's respiratory pattern most likely has which of the following pathologies?
    A. Diabetic ketoacidosis
    B. Ischemic Stroke
    C. Hemorrhagic stroke
    D. Brain trauma

    Answer
    A. Correct. Diabetic ketoacidosis is associated with Kussmaul's breathing pattern.
    B. Incorrect. Ischemic stroke would more likely exhibit an apneustic or biots-breathing pattern.
    C. Incorrect. Hemorrhagic stroke would more likely exhibit an apneustic or biots-breathing pattern.
    D. Incorrect. Brain trauma would more likely exhibit an apneustic or biots-breathing pattern.

20. Pneumothorax is suspected in a mechanically ventilated patient in the ICU. The patient is on assist control mode and has a size 8.0 ETT secured at 22cm at the lip. The patient is hemodynamically stable. What should the therapist recommend NEXT?
    A. Arterial blood gas
    B. Withdraw the ETT 2 cm
    C. Portable chest X-ray
    D. Switch to pressure control ventilation

    Answer
    A. Incorrect. An ABG will neither confirm a pneumothorax, nor treat one.
    B. Incorrect. There is no evidence the ETT is in the wrong position. In addition, withdrawing the ETT may cause a loss of the patient's airway.
    C. Correct. The patient is stable, which allows time to confirm the presence of a pneumothorax.
    D. Incorrect. Pressure control ventilation will not treat a pneumothorax and may under ventilate the patient, due to the high intrathoracic pressures associated with a pneumothorax.

I really hope you liked this book. Let's be honest; I hope you loved it! But, just in case you didn't, I'd love to hear from you. Tell me what could make this book better. What do you feel I may have missed?

Here is my personal email: respprograms@gmail.com. Let me know what you think. Tell me the good, the bad, and the horrible. This will only help me make better products for YOU and, other respiratory therapists/students out there.

If this book met your expectations and is helpful to you, please leave a review on the Amazon sales page here: http://www.amazon.com/dp/B01BM0AK3S.

I'm hard at work on the next book in this series. To get a free preview of the next book before it is released, sign up to my subscriber newsletter at www.respiratorytherapyprograms.com.

References

Heur, A. J., Scanlan, C. L. *Wilkins' Clinical Assessment in Respiratory Care*. 2014. Mosby. 7th edition.

Kacmarek, R. M., Stoller, J. K., Heuer, A. J., *Egan's Fundamentals of Respiratory Care*. Elsevier, 2013. 10th edition.

www.ingramcontent.com/pod-product-compliance
Lightning Source LLC
Chambersburg PA
CBHW040850180526
45159CB00001B/375